269
amazing
s e x
games

Hugh de Beer

SOURCEBOOKS CASABLANCA™
AN IMPRINT OF SOURCEBOOKS, INC.®
NAPERVILLE, ILLINOIS

Published by Sourcebooks, Inc.
P.O. Box 4410, Naperville, Illinois 60567-4410
(630) 961-3900
fax: (630) 961-2168
www.sourcebooks.com

ISBN-10: 1-4022-0352-7
ISBN-13: 978-1-4022-0352-7

Printed and bound in the United States of America
CPI 10 9 8 7 6 5 4 3 2 1

contents

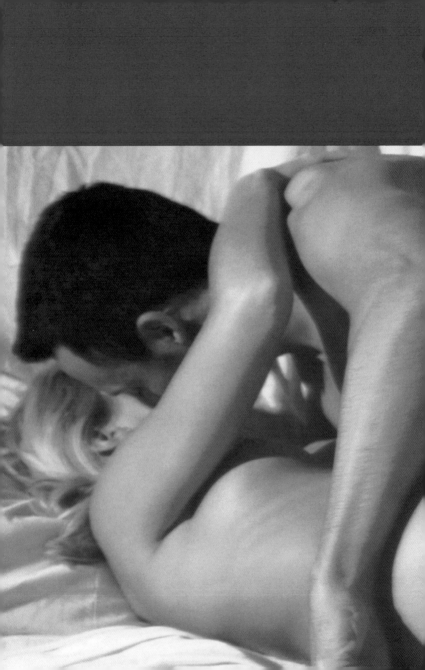

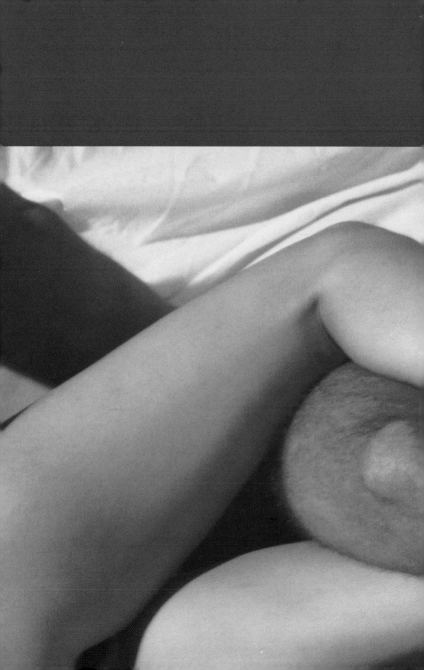

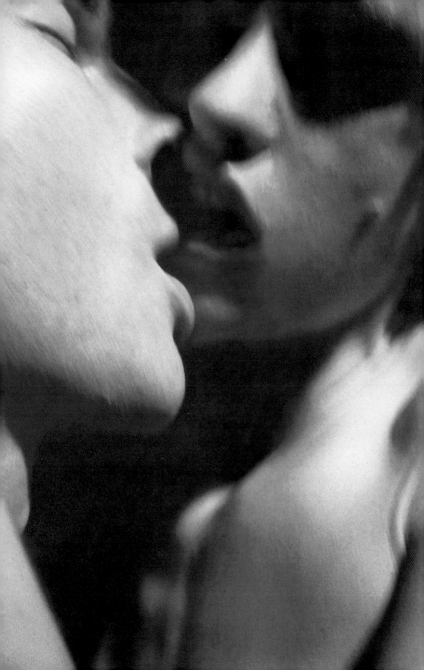

ONE | eat, drink, and be merry

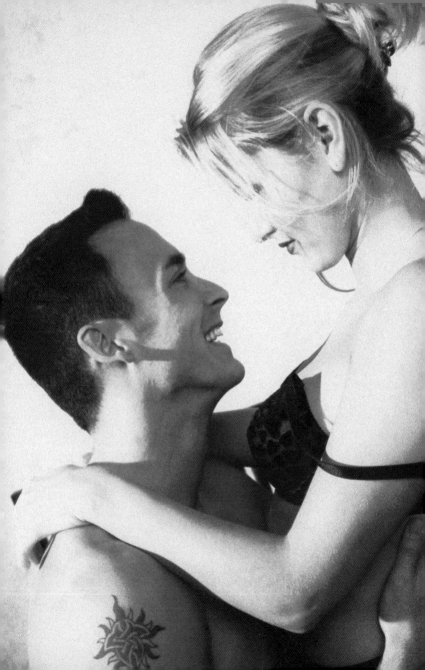

eating out

| | Next time you're out for dinner, write sexual suggestions on your napkins and swap with each other.

2 | Every time you have sex, place $10 in a safe place. When you have enough money, spend it on a romantic dinner.

3 | When you find yourself at a restaurant table with a long tablecloth, use your feet to bring your lover to orgasm. Don't stop when the waiter's there.

4 | Pretend you're on your honeymoon (married or not, engaged or not—don't make it significant) and can't get enough of each other. Feed each other by hand, link arms and drink champagne, kiss and fondle. Who knows; if you convince those around you, they may buy you dessert!

5 | Before you go out, write a steamy, suggestive, anonymous note. When you get to the restaurant, slip it to the waiter to deliver to your partner during the course of the evening. Observe their reaction and ask about the content of the note. The rest is up to you.

come and get it

6 Feed your blindfolded lover a special meal you have prepared. If they can correctly guess what they're eating, they win a full body massage.

7 Dress up like a waiter/waitress and tease each other while serving a favorite meal.

8 Your lover blindfolds you and places some food on your naked body. If you can guess what it is, you win and your lover eats it off. If not, your lover can make a wish and ask you to carry it out.

9 Make a list of ten ingredients that make for great sex.

10 Plan a menu for lust. Appetizers might include taking the phone off the hook, putting on sexy music, and dancing naked in the living room; the main course might include a bottle of good wine and massage oil; dessert might involve chocolate and sweet words.

11 Have a food fight in the nude so you can clean up later with your mouths and tongues.

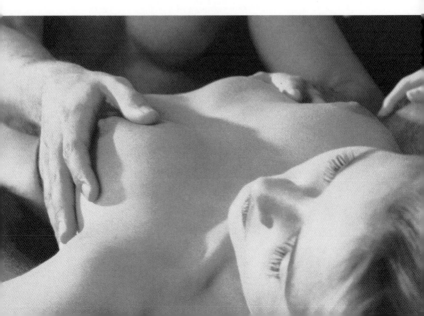

passion fruit

12 Take a luscious ripe cherry and stroke it slowly around your partner's lips. Place the polished surface against your own lips, then take a nibble from it before popping it into their mouth.

13 Prepare your favorite fruit and arrange it artfully over your lover's naked body before eating it off.

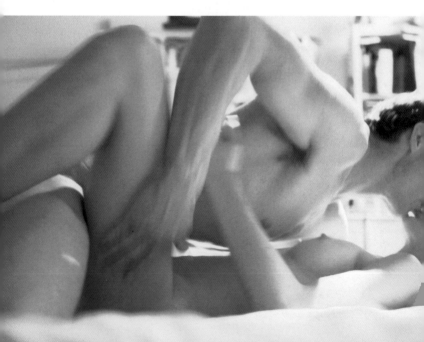

14 Take turns rubbing a ripe, warm, juicy orange or mango all over your lover's body. Lick off as much as you can. The one to do the best job cleaning off the other wins a sexual favor of their choice.

15 Talk about something erotic you'd like to do with fruit (or a vegetable). Go to the grocery store and consider the possibilities.

16 Get a collection of fruit juices—strawberry, orange, pineapple, mango, guava, peach, apricot, blackberry—and have your lover close their eyes. Cover their lips with juice, then lick them clean. Try the flavors one by one and have your lover guess each fruit.

icecapades

17 Pass an ice cube from mouth to mouth. The first to drop it has to perform any sexual act the winner wishes.

18 Dust talcum powder all over your partner's body. Take an ice cube and use it to make patterns through the powder. The feeling of cold on hot skin is sensational.

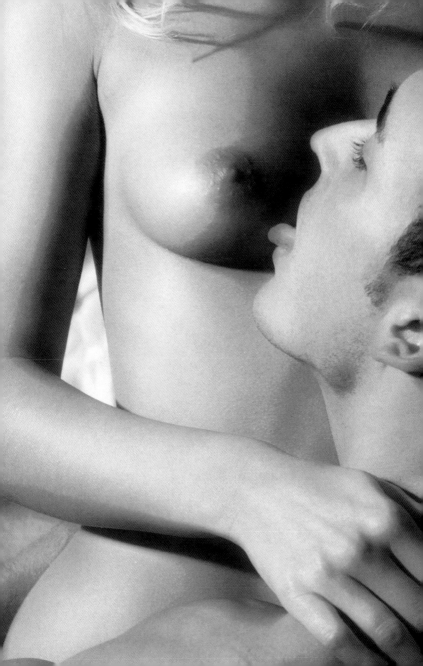

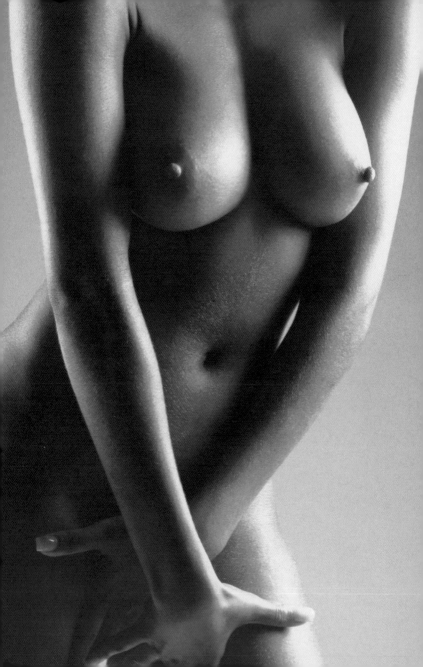

foreplay feast

Work up your lover's anticipation during the day with a campaign of erotic suggestions sent along in their lunch or briefcase.

19 Send chocolates with a sexy note to your lover.

20 Make sandwiches and include a photo of yourself naked in the wrapping.

21 Phone your lover at lunchtime and tell them what part of their body you would like to eat.

22 Tear a page from an adult magazine or lingerie catalog, fold it up, and put it in their pocket (be sure this won't get them fired).

23 Tuck a banana or mango into their lunch with suggestions for how they can enjoy it.

desirable desserts

24 Make a plaster cast mold of your lover's genitals and cast chocolate statues to be eaten before, during, or after sex.

25 Make a sundae on your lover's genitals or breasts using your favorite sauces, fruit, and whipped cream. Decorate with nuts or sprinkles, and don't forget the cherry. Then dig in.

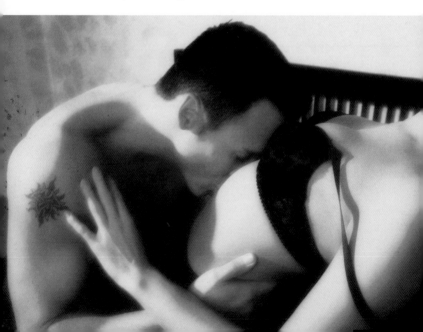

drinking games

26 Invent a new soft drink or cocktail and name it after your lover.

27 Place an old blanket on the ground and have your lover lie on it. Pour your favorite champagne into your lover's navel and over their stomach. Try to drink it before it hits the blanket.

28 Fill water pistols with wine and squirt each other before licking clean.

29 Organize a naked cocktail party for two and use different parts of the body to hold the drinks.

30 Have your man use his penis to stir your drink, then place it in your mouth so you don't waste a drop.

31 Sitting in a cocktail lounge, I could sense someone looking at me. As I casually turned my head, an attractive figure caught my eye. My date was now half an hour late, and I was getting impatient. I forgot my troubles, however, when the gorgeous stranger now looking my way gave me a wink and suggestively moistened their lips with their tongue. The stranger held up a glass of champagne and toasted me. How should I respond? Should I hold out for my date, get up and introduce myself, or wait for the stranger to approach? The bartender served me another drink...

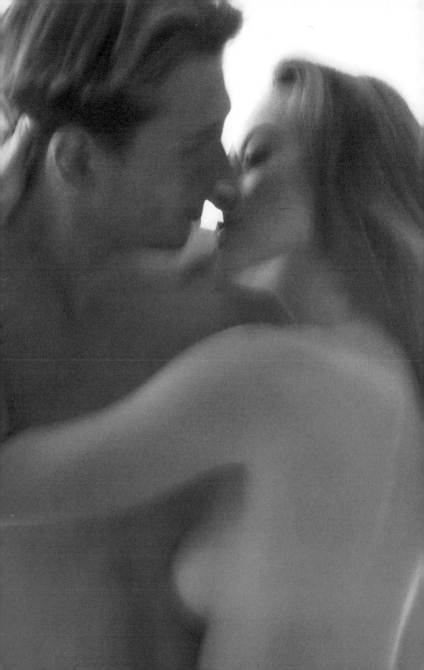

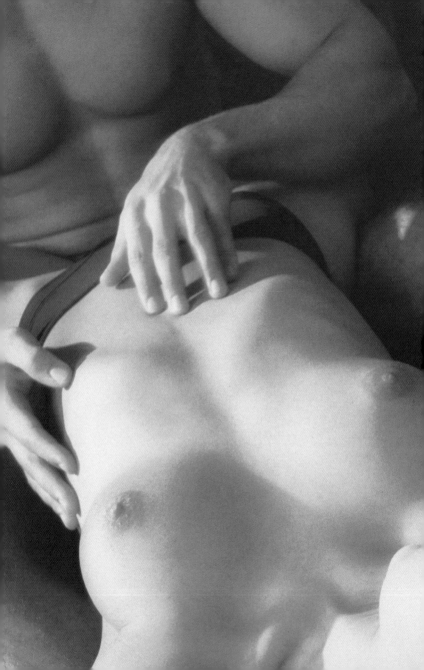

two | playing the field

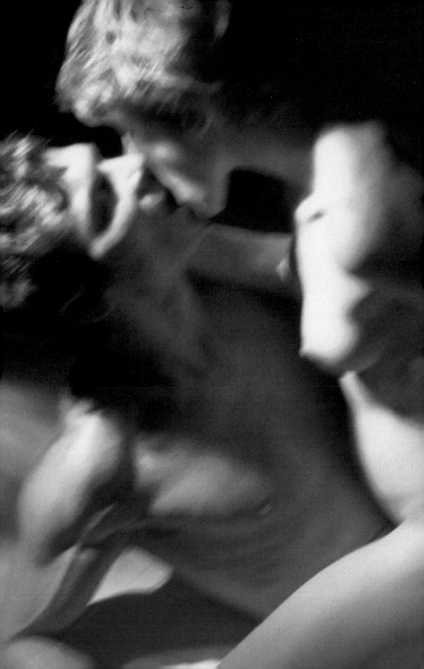

sexercise

3 2   Watch each other doing stretching exercises naked, or scantily clothed, before having sex.

3 3   Try having sex on a "Fitball."

3 4   Incorporate your favorite sports equipment and clothing into your next lovemaking session.

3 5   Play naked touch football together.

hitting the mat

36 Place a large sheet of plastic on the floor. Cover your body and your lover's body with oil and have a wrestling match.

37 Naked, and with your bodies covered in oil, sit on the floor back-to-back with your partner. Link elbows and try to stand up together.

38 Sumo-wrestle on the bed.

39 Sex is a team sport for two, so develop a win-win strategy.

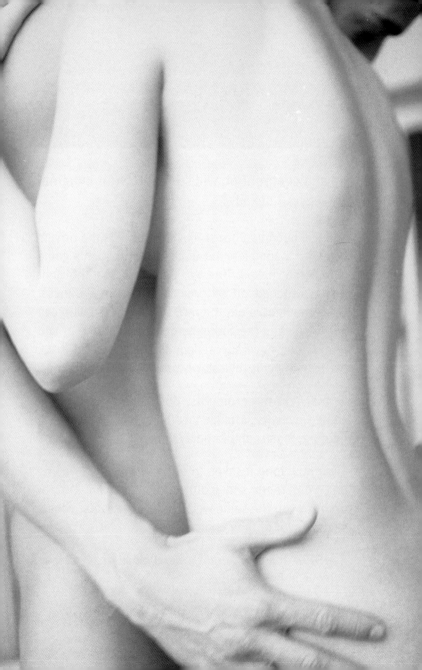

setting records

Challenges and competition will stimulate your imagination as well as your sex life.

40 You will need two boxes. Each of you fills the other's box with a complete set of clothing. Start this game completely naked. The go signal will be the light being switched off to provide complete darkness. Once the light is off, the race begins to see who can get dressed in the complete outfit. When one of you thinks they have succeeded, switch the lights back on. The winner is then slowly undressed by their lover.

41 In the next three months, don't make love in the same way twice. Change locations, positions, speed, lighting, music, and foreplay games.

42 Time how long it takes to undress your lover using just your teeth and mouth. Then let your partner undress you the same way. Whoever's fastest wins a sexual favor of their choice.

43 See how many different sexual positions you can achieve in five minutes.

44 Keep track of how many simultaneous orgasms you have in a week, a month, or a year.

45 In three minutes, write down as many positive aspects of your partner's lovemaking techniques as you can. When time's up, compare and discuss lists.

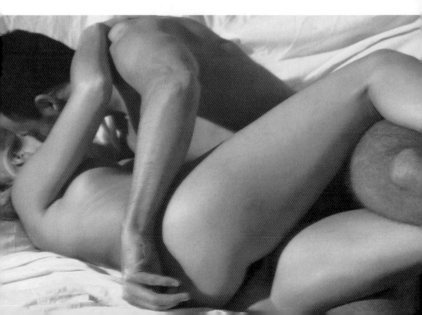

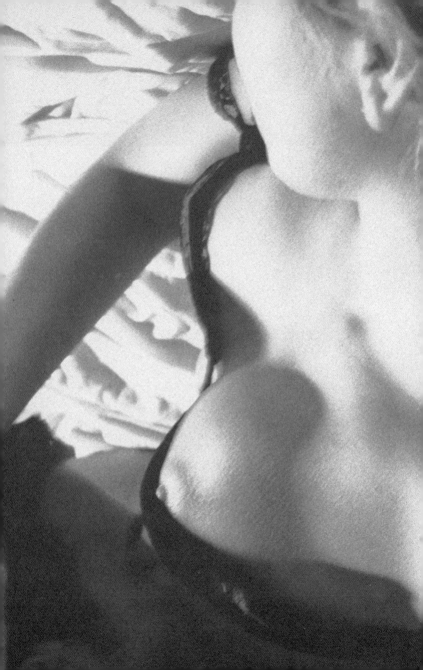

a tease a day
keeps the blues away

Be a tease, but know the boundaries. For instance, if your lover really hates being tickled, that's off-limits.

46 Get into the "69" position and massage each other without touching the genitals.

47 Use a vibrator to stimulate all over your partner's body. Carefully work very close to, but don't touch, the genital area or the nipples. When your lover is driven completely wild with desire and cannot lie still anymore, you have won.

48 Take a condom out of its packet and use your imagination to devise games with it. Keep in the spirit of devilment and fun. Be careful not to be too hard on the condom if you're going to use it afterwards. If you're thinking of tying your lover to the bed using several condoms, be mindful of safe sex and use a fresh one in the appropriate location.

49 You could try stretching the condom and flicking your lover's bottom with it. Tie inflated condoms to each of your ankles. On the given word, try to burst each other's condoms. The one who pops the condom first is the winner and has their favorite sexual pleasure acted out.

50 Standing naked facing your partner, hold an inflated condom between your stomachs. Without using your hands, attempt to:
- Move around the room.
- Move the condom up to your chins.

- Turn around so the condom is held between your backs.
- Lower yourself to the floor with the condom held between your backs.

5 | Blow up a condom and play:
- Tennis
- Volleyball
- Hockey

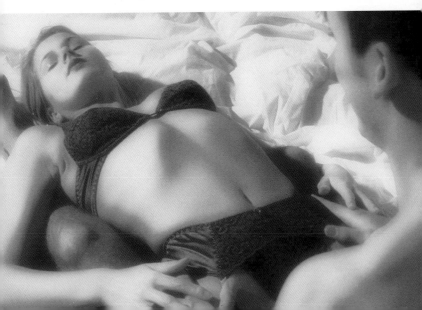

don't lose your marbles

52 Place as many marbles as possible under your fitted bed sheet before having sex. Also try...
- Ping-pong balls
- Golf balls
- Blown-up condoms

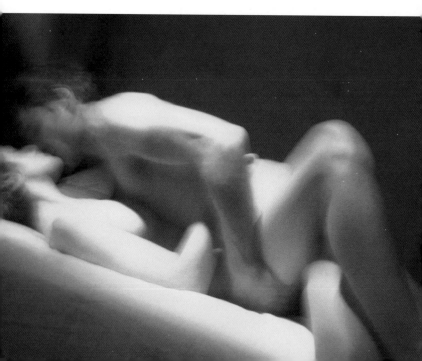

53 Sitting naked behind your lover on the floor, move around the room in unison. This is a great way to strengthen the butt.

54 Massage your lover's feet while they read erotic material aloud.

55 Work out sexual activities you can do with the following: eight rubber bands, soap, and a bicycle pump.

56 Make love as though you were both seventy years old. Then, as though you were both seventeen years old.

57 Have sex in the snow. You may need to keep your hats on.

58 You go to a professional football game and get separated from your friends. As you wander around the stadium trying to find the way back to your seat, you accidentally find your-self in one of the locker rooms. It appears empty, with the exception of a solitary figure lying on one of the benches. You move forward for a closer look...

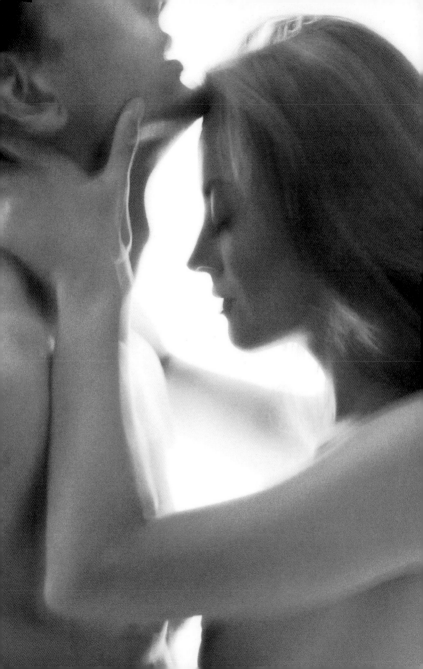

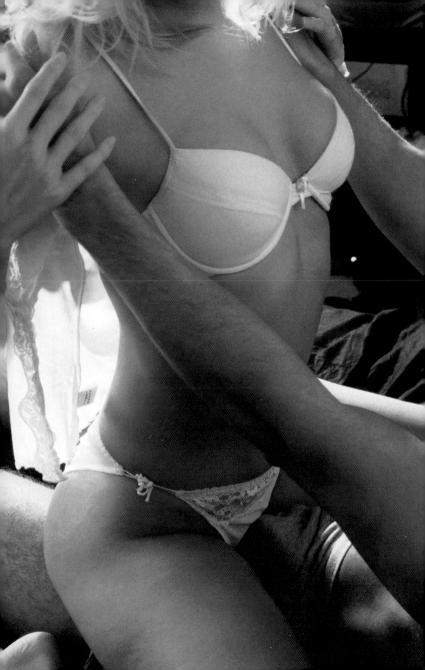

THREE | casino consummation

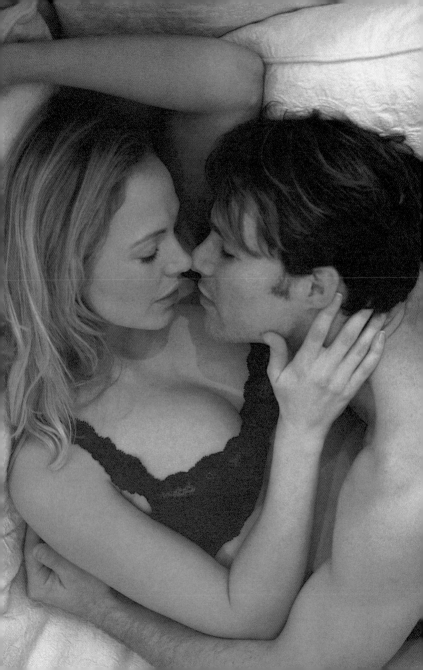

59 Bet on anything—which of two ants will reach the end of the counter first, for example. The winner then picks a number between 1 and 269 in this book as a prize.

60 Auction off pieces of clothing that you are wearing for sexual favors.

61 Auction off sexual favors for getting jobs done around the house.

62 Toss a coin to see who takes the dominant position.

hat tricks

63 Make a number of cards with famous lovers (Antony and Cleopatra, Superman and Lois Lane, Popeye and Olive Oyl). Place the cards in a hat and randomly select a card. Have sex in the way you think the famous pair would.

64 Wear different types of hats when you have sex.

Write romantic and sensuous actions (such as the following) on separate strips of paper and place in a hat. Each day take out one strip and perform the action. When you have completed an action, stick the strip on the fridge.

65 Book a room in a motel and take a picnic basket and some wine with you. Put the "Do not disturb" sign on the door and let them wonder.

66 Go to your partner's workplace and find a safe place for a "quickie."

67 Buy your lover something sexy and make a date to enjoy it.

68 Send your partner their favorite flowers with a steamy message on the card.

69 Give your lover oral sex while they sleep.

70 Plan a whole day devoted to sex.

71 Have sex fully clothed.

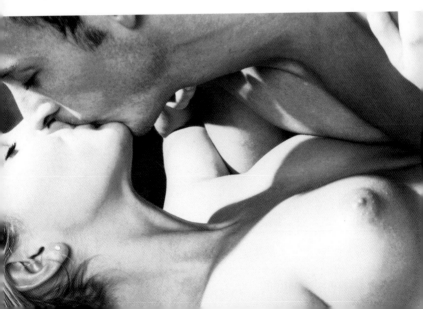

Write answers to the following questions on strips of paper. Place the strips of paper into a hat and then choose one. Read the strip out loud and enact the method prescribed on the paper.

72 Favorite sexual invitation?

73 Favorite lovemaking position?

74 Favorite dirty talk?

75 Favorite sexual technique?

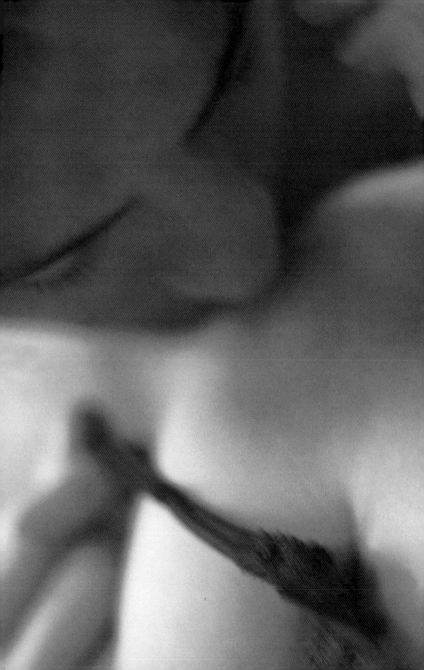

snake eyes

76 Select six different places where you can make love. Assign each place a number from 1 to 6, and roll a die for your selection. These should be previously unexplored places in the home, such as on top of the washing machine or under the bed.

77 Select six different times during the day to have sex. Assign the times a number from 1 to 6 and roll a die to schedule your next adventure.

78 Strip Dice: The players take turns throwing a pair of dice. Each number on the dice represents an article of clothing to be removed, as listed below. The winner is the one who gets all the clothing off their partner first.

2: Tie or scarf	8: Dress or skirt
3: Socks/stockings	9: Bra or undershirt
4: Underpants	10: Belt
5: Shirt	11: Watch or bracelet
6: Pants	12: Necklace or chain
7: Jacket	

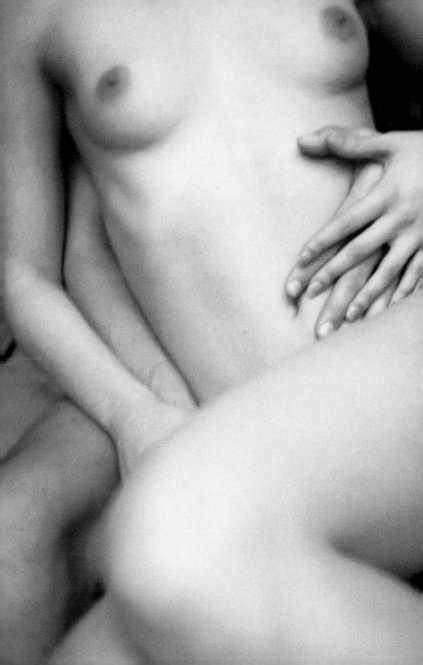

79 Sexy Numbers: Each number on one of the die is to represent a different part of the body while each number on the other die is to represent an action. Use the dice to make up your own games.

1: Lips
2: Breasts
3: Neck
4: Genitals
5: Bottom
6: Feet

1: Licking
2: Sucking
3: Nibbling
4: Stroking
5: Kissing
6: Massaging

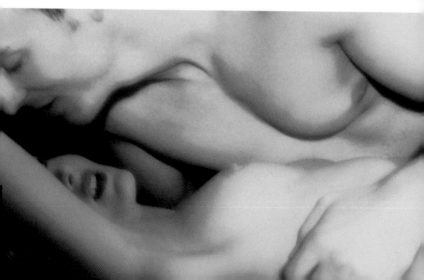

80 Roll a die; the highest score begins. Each number on the die represents one of the scenarios below. Out loud, complete the scenario that corresponds with the number you rolled.

1: I had no choice but to lie back and enjoy the warmth of those hands caressing my body...

2: I had never been involved in a trio, and I wasn't going to let this opportunity pass...

3: Waiting outside my apartment for a taxi, I couldn't help but notice through a bedroom window a couple making love...

4: Traveling home on the train late at night, I noticed the only other occupant, a gorgeous stranger, was looking straight at me...

5: There I was, stretched out naked on the bed, with my hands and feet tied. The door opened and my dominant partner entered, wearing...

6: The first time I made love was...

pick a card, any card

Make up your own personal card deck of simple foreplay ideas—a great help for those times when you feel lacking in imagination. Cut up card stock or manila file folders into 2" x 3" rectangles and write up your favorites. You can each draw three and perform the actions in sequence, or make up your own card games. You may also want to have picture cards, or some designating time periods. Here are some for starters.

8 1 | Nibble behind.

8 2 Lick breasts.

8 3 Massage toes.

8 4 Blindfold partner.

8 5 Blindfold self.

8 6 Perform striptease.

87 Stroke hands.

88 Talk dirty.

89 Suck fingers.

90 Standing up.

91 Dance naked.

92 Describe genitals.

93 Massage face.

94 Undress partner.

95 You sweep into the casino dressed in the sexi-est, most elegant clothes imaginable, and all heads turn to admire you as you walk by. At the far end of the room is a figure straight out of a James Bond movie, and they're waiting for you. As the two of you win at roulette time after time, the sexual tension mounts. Finally, you leave the bright lights of the hot room and step out onto a starlit balcony in the cool night air...

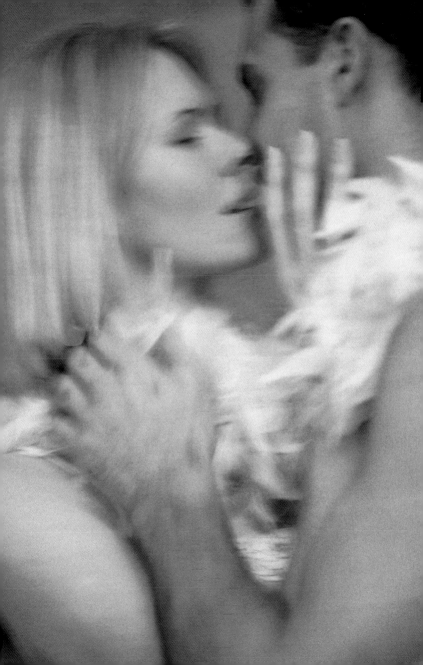

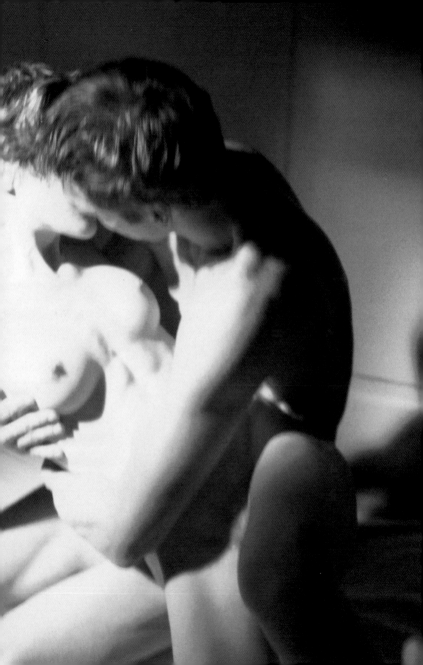

FOUR | the art of seduction

body art

Body painting is still as colorful and captivating as it was centuries ago. Women in Ancient Greece used body paints on their breasts to lure curious males. Sophisticates of the European Renaissance courts used heavy red rouge for sexual attraction.

96 Use watercolor paints to decorate your partner's breasts. You may wish to take a photo of your artwork. When you have finished, wash the paint off with warm water and a soft washcloth.

97 Spend a little time thinking about what design you will paint onto your partner's body. You might only want to paint the top half of the body, the bottom, the front, or the back. When you have decided what your masterpiece is going to be like, you both undress and start painting each other at the same time. Take time and care over your human canvas. When you have finished and are happy with your artwork, take a photo. Don't forget to sign your painting.

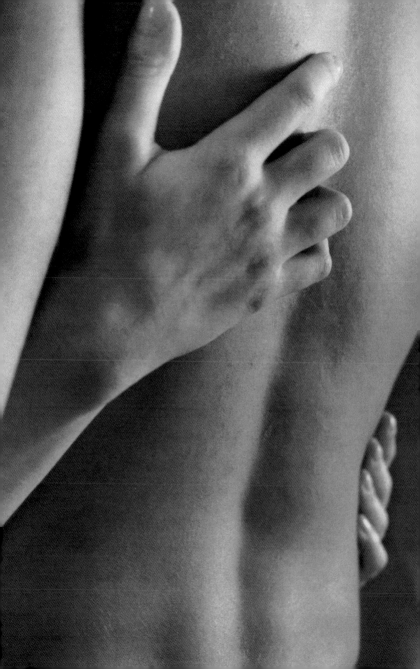

art class

98 Spread large sheets of white paper on the floor. Splash different colors of acrylic paint over your naked bodies and roll over the paper together. Frame the best painting.

99 Learn to make plaster casts of different parts of your lover's body. Try to end up with a complete life-size model.

100 Set yourself up with a canvas, several soft paint brushes, and body paints. Paint a picture of your lover's whole body or just areas of your lover that fascinate you, such as a hand, foot, or cheek. Frame the finished painting and hang it in your bedroom.

make beautiful music together

Hot music such as ragtime, blues, boogie-woogie, and jazz originated in the notorious sporting clubs of the New Orleans red light district. The word jazz itself was thought to have been derived from the African American word "jizz," which is supposed to imply exercise in a horizontal position. Pianist and composer Clarence Williams laid claim to being the originator of jazz after hearing a woman comment on his music, saying, "Oh jazz me baby" with sexual overtones.

101 Put on some hot jazz and get close to your partner, then move your body to the music. Don't worry how you look.

102 The name "swing" is derived from the ladies who could swing their bosoms and the men who jiggled their assets. Go out with your lover and do some dirty dancing. Let's face it, "It don't mean a thing when you ain't got that swing."

103 Design your own erotic sound tracks. Select musical pieces that you associate with certain moods, such as hard rock for a wild romp, or classical music for a sophisticated evening.

104 This game can be played by randomly selecting songs off the radio, or using your own CD collection. What songs do you associate with:

• Foreplay (Appetizer)
• Sex (Main course)
• Afterplay (Dessert)

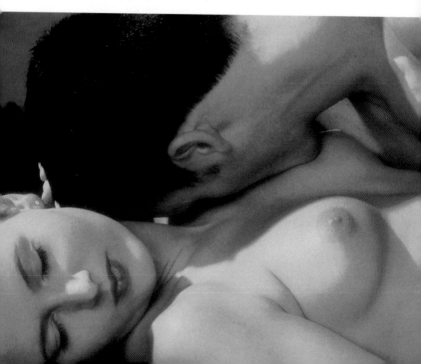

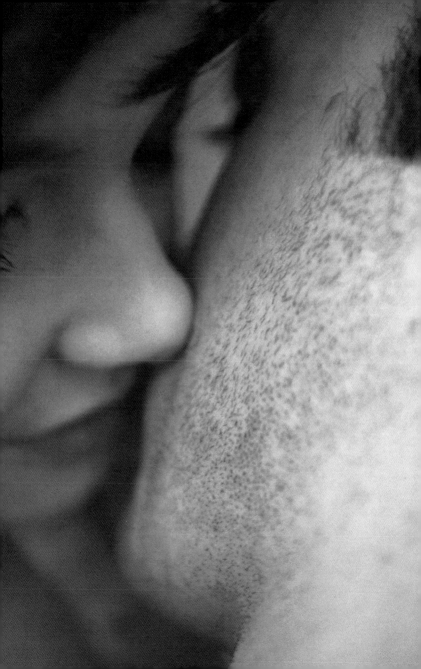

picture perfect

105 Make an X-rated photo album of intimate moments you share. If necessary, stage or reenact scenes to get just the pictures you want.

106 Take photographs of your partner in various stages of undress and frame the montage.

107 Cut out images from magazines to make up a collage of your lover. Design a "Coat of Arms" that would best describe your relationship together.

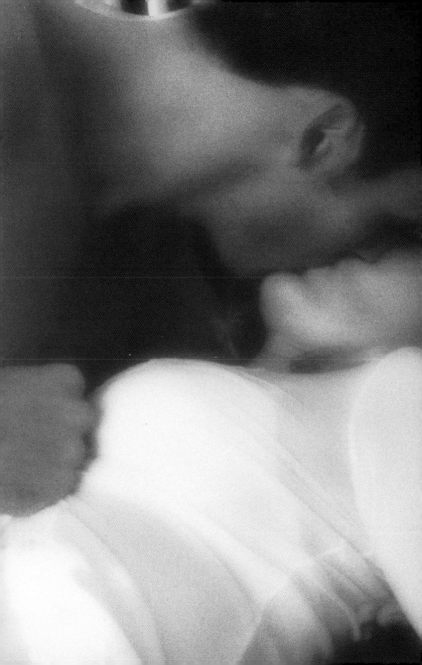

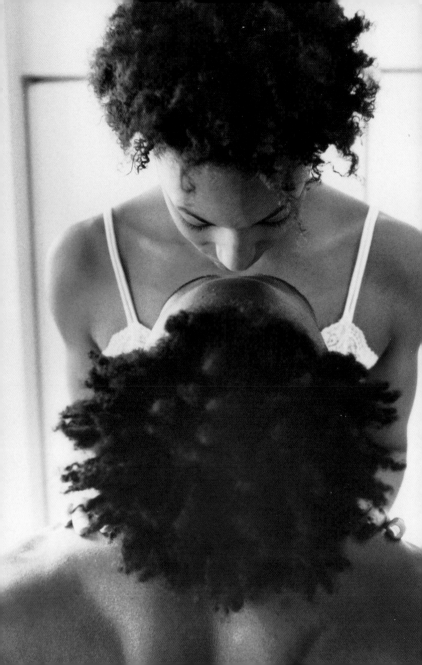

puzzle pieces

108 Buy an erotic jigsaw puzzle and put it together with your lover.

109 Take one picture of your lover and one picture of you. Cut them into jigsaw puzzle pieces that are tricky to recognize on their own. Mix up both sets of photos to make the puzzle more difficult to unravel. The winner is the one that can put together both puzzles in the shortest amount of time.

110 Write an X-rated love note and cut it into simple jigsaw pieces. Put the pieces in an envelope and mail it to your lover.

scrapbook sex

Instead of just a photo album of vacations and birthday parties, create a "Best Sex" scrapbook or chart. Update it as appropriate. This is a great way to remember the intimate moments you've shared.

||| Locations and place
Best session in bed...
Best session in a car...
Best session outside...
Best unusual place...

||2 Health and fitness
Most athletic session...
Wildest...
Most romantic session...
Most interesting position...

||3 Times
The first time together...
The most memorable session...
The funniest session...
The anniversary...

114 Techniques
The most bizarre...
The best position...
The most loving...
The highest energy...

115 Toys
Best video...
Most erotic reading material...
Best body lotion...
Best sex toys...

116 Wish list
For the bedroom...
Toys...
Gifts...
Other...

117 Position
Best dominant...
Best submissive...
Most intense orgasm...
Most relaxed...

118 Personal best
Fill in as appropriate.

119 You've been living in Paris, but times are hard. You're forced to take work posing as a nude model for an art class. It's strenuous work. One of the most difficult things is mingling with the perfect bodies of the other models without letting your arousal show. One day, as the class is breaking up and the students are putting away their materials, you feel a hand on your arm...

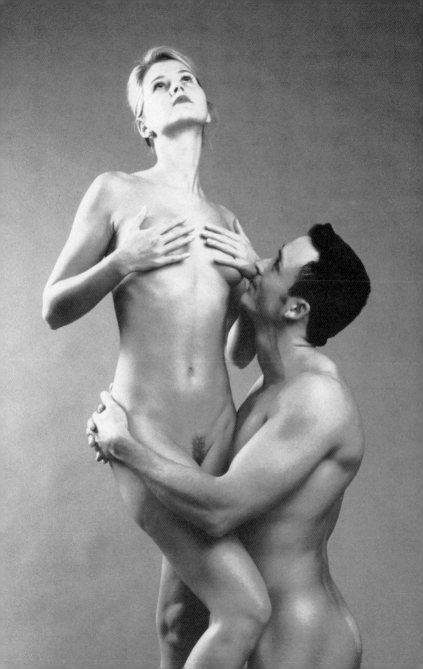

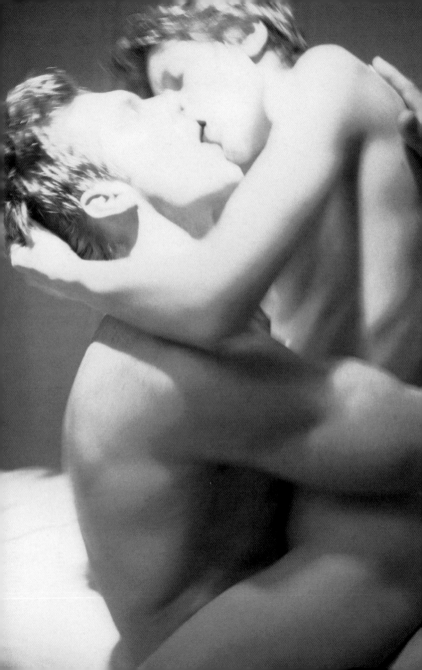

FIVE | lights, camera, action!

for the exhibitionist in you

120 Reenact a steamy scene from a movie that turns you on. If it works for you it is sure to turn your lover on.

121 Make your own porno movie together.

122 Devise and make a thirty-second television ad to sell your sexual assets.

123 Play fantasy dress-up for each other. Try roles like nurses, soldiers, prostitutes, gigolos, pirates, actors, etc.

124 Present your lover with sexual awards similar to the Oscars.

125 Videotape yourselves talking together, kissing, danc- ing, doing the dishes, playing cards, cuddling, watch- ing television. Watch the tape and observe your body language, the way you touch. Share what you like (or don't like).

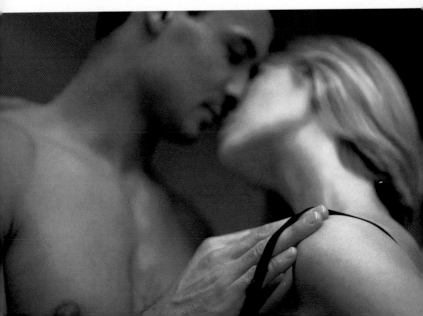

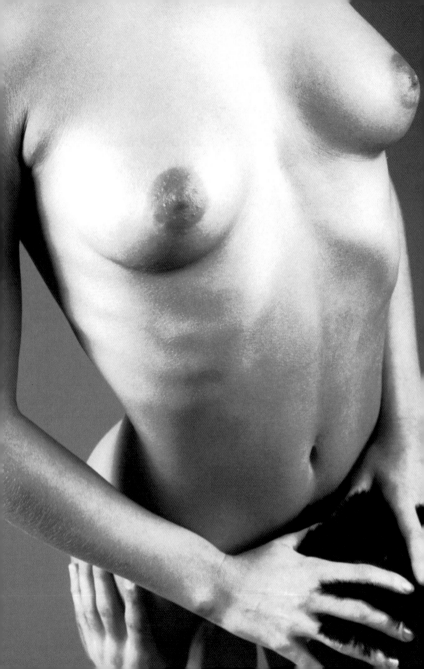

126 Sit in front of a mirror naked and draw a picture of your genitals. Make a note of the areas that are sensitive to the touch. Give it to your lover as your own personal sex manual.

127 Position a mirror so that your lover can watch as you kiss and caress their genitals.

128 Have "fright night" watching scary movies. Jump each other's bones during the scary bits.

129 Watch a "beginner's guide to sex" video together. Rewrite the script to incorporate details from your own first sexual experience.

130 Write the titles of six erotic videos on slips of paper. Close your eyes and select one to watch tonight.

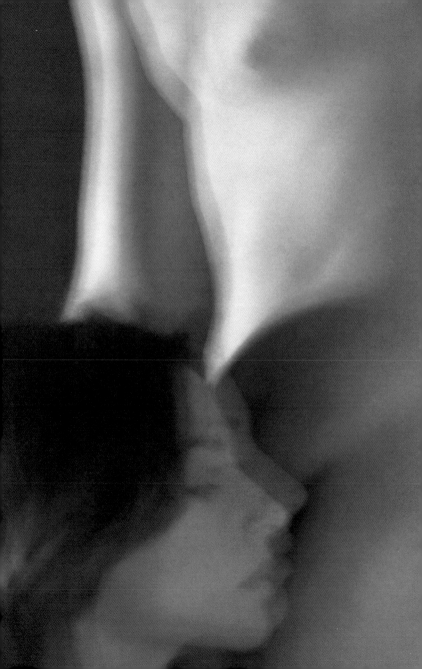

role with it

Role-playing is a fun way to be adventurous and push sexual boundaries.

131 Sex Therapist and Patient: Toss a coin to see who takes the roles of Sex Therapist and Patient. The Therapist has to go somewhere private to be able to answer the call of the Patient. The Patient rings the Therapist and pretends to ask for advice on how to please their partner. The Therapist goes into great detail describing a way to please their partner.

132 Master/Mistress and Slave: Toss a coin to see who takes the role of Master or Mistress. Once the roles have been established, the Slave has to carry out every action required of them without question.

133 Confessor and Priest/Priestess: Toss a coin to see who takes the roles of Confessor and Priest/Priestess. Set up two chairs with a sheet or blanket hanging between them. The Confessor says: "Forgive me, for I have sinned." The Priest/Priestess is to question the Confessor in order to get to the bottom of the matter. After the Confessor confesses to any given sin, the Priest/Priestess replies, "For your sins you are to perform the following foreplay actions..."

134 This is a role-play game where you select an identity of someone real or imaginary (actor, politician, historical figure, etc.). Don't tell each other who you're being—your partner must guess. Once you have both selected an identity, you play the role of that person. Now you have five minutes in which to seduce your partner. The seduction cannot be consummated until you have both successfully guessed each other's roles or the time runs out, in which case you start again with different characters.

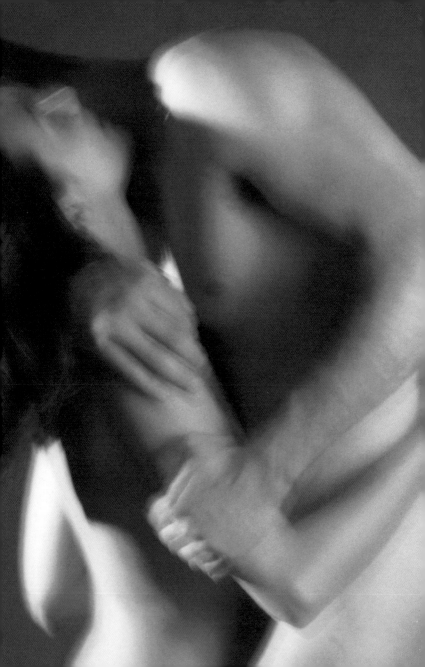

finish the fantasy

135 You've always dreamed of being a famous actor and you hurry to the audition with great anticipation. You find the address and wonder why you have to go up three flights of stairs to the studio. The door is opened by a tall, handsome black man who introduces himself as the director. There's nothing in the room but a video camera, a bucket of chilled champagne, and a bed occupied by two beautiful women, one blonde and one Asian...

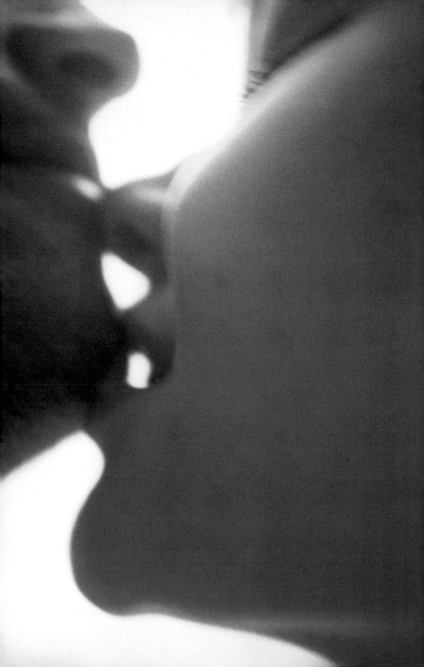

six | word play

136 Do a word-association test with each other using words such as: love, foreplay, sex, music, politics.

137 Create a crossword puzzle with words that show your feelings for your lover. Be as explicit as you like. Then see if they can solve the puzzle.

138 Play X-rated Scrabble. Award one point per letter used, so "foreplay" scores eight, while "orgasm" scores six—and the person who can spell "cunnilingus" will probably win!

139 List the letters of the alphabet down the side of a piece of paper. For each letter, write something that describes what your lover does to turn you on. For example: A = His sensuous Aroma turns me on. B = I love her beautiful Breasts.

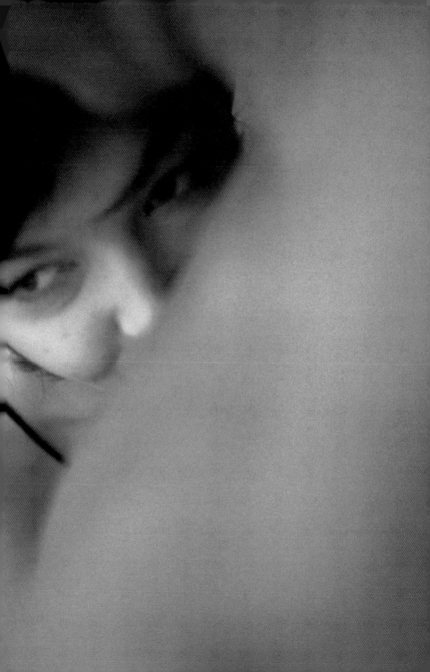

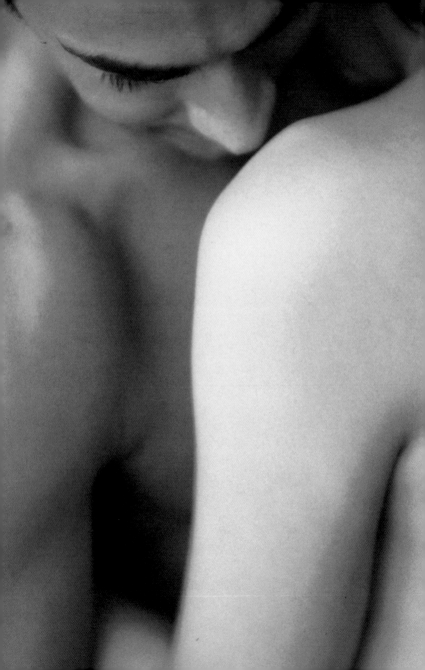

literary prowess

140 Memorize a Shakespeare sonnet and recite it while making love.

141 Role-play the balcony scene from Romeo and Juliet.

142 Read your lover an erotic bedtime story.

143 Read old love poems your partner sent you on anniversaries. Try to reenact those occasions on rainy days.

144 Buy two sex books or magazines and underline things of interest. Swap titles and see if you understand why your partner underlined what they did. After you have finished both, discuss.

story time

145 Recall the first time you made love and tell the full story to your lover, describing how you truly felt.

146 Create an erotic adventure story with your lover. You start by making up the first sentence. Your lover continues with the next. Go on until your fictional story has reached a happy ending. Then act out the story to make the fantasy a reality.

147 Describe a sexual fantasy to your lover. Then ask them to retell it in as much detail as they can remember.

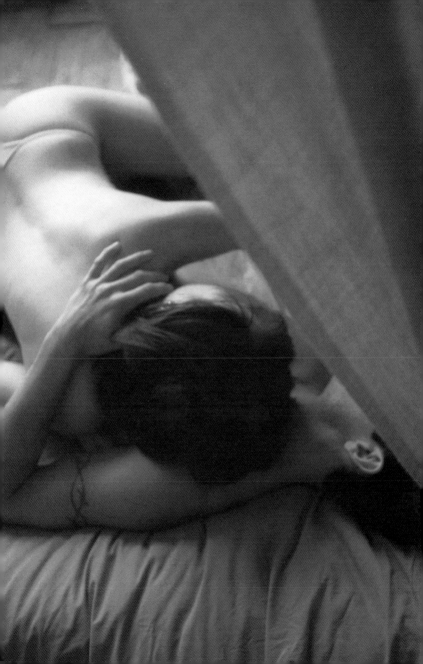

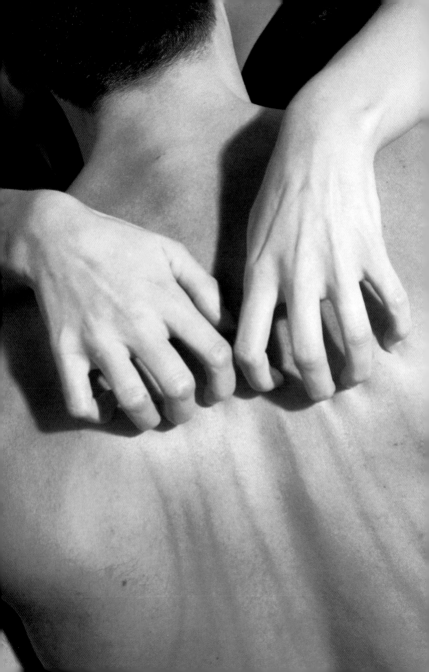

xxx creative writing

148 Write about the most enjoyable orgasm you have achieved. Note the time of the day, place, and person you shared the orgasm with. What made it special? Could you recreate the exact circumstances again? If it was a moment you shared with your current lover, send them a copy in a thank-you note.

149 Keep a diary of your lovemaking and read it nightly with your lover.

150 Write about your most adventurous sexual escapades and send to a magazine—you might get published!

| 5 | Novel Sex: You will need a piece of paper and a pencil. Read the first question and write your answer, then fold the top of the paper forward to cover your words. Pass the sheet to your partner for them to write the next answer. Again fold the paper, and continue until all the questions are answered. Unfold the page and read your story. Now try to make up your own questions to develop a story.

1. Use one or two adjectives to describe your lover.

2. Write the name of a female you respect.

3. Write the word "met" and an adjective to describe your first sexual experience.

4. Write the name of a male you can identify with.

5. Write the words "in the" and the name of a place where you feel comfortable.

6. Finish this sentence: "I can't say no when…"

7. Complete the following: "Let's play…"

8. Do you prefer to be in a crowd or alone?

9. What's sexually adventurous for you?

10. What time of day do you like to make love?

11. Would you rather be fully dressed, partially dressed, or naked?

12. How do you ask your partner for sex?

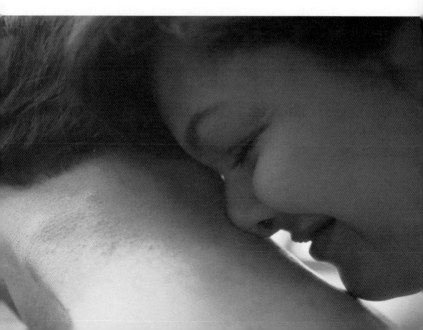

you've got mail

Use the following tips to carry on a secret affair with your lover. Don't discuss your letters, except in your written reply. Only write positive things.

152 Buy your own special stationery and spray with a signature scent.

153 Write a one-page letter and send it to your lover. Don't type the letter; it's more personal if it's handwritten. Write the letter as neatly as possible and proofread before sending.

154 Send the letter by post; don't hand-deliver.

155 Make it a rule that you have to respond within a few days of receiving your letter.

156 Use your letters to fantasize—if you are shy, describe yourself as outgoing, if you wear bright clothes, say you wear plain clothes, etc.

157 After a few months of letter writing, you might like to "meet." Plan it as though a pair of pen pals are meeting for the first time. You may want to keep the letter affair going for years *without* meeting.

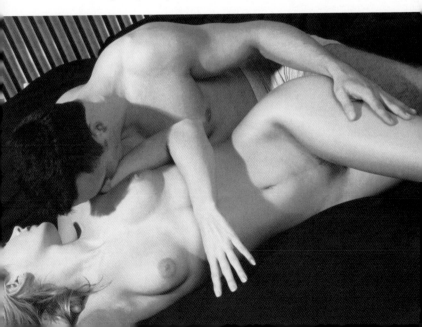

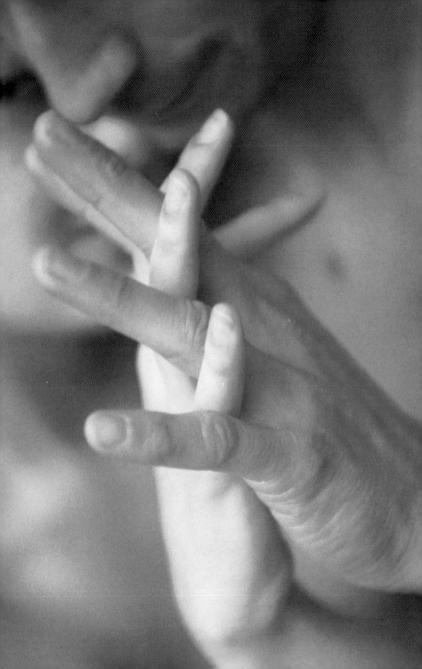

seriously sexy

158 Spend some time with your lover drawing up an adventurous ten-point sexual plan in the same way that you'd draw up a business or investment plan.

159 Design a two-day sex plan that you can carry out over the weekend.

160 Just for fun, write and negotiate a sexual contract that will please you both.

161 Make a list of ten sexual commandments you both have to live by. Update regularly.

sex calendar

162 Take erotic photographs of you and your partner and create a sex calendar. Write in appointments with your own erotic ideas.

163 Circle days on the calendar when you "have to" make love. No excuses.

164 Circle days on the calendar when you will make love in different rooms in the house. List the room, time, place, and method.

165 Circle days on the calendar when you will give your lover an orgasm without intercourse.

166 Circle days on the calendar when you will make love in different positions.

167 Circle days on the calendar when you will perform foreplay only.

168 Circle special romantic days.

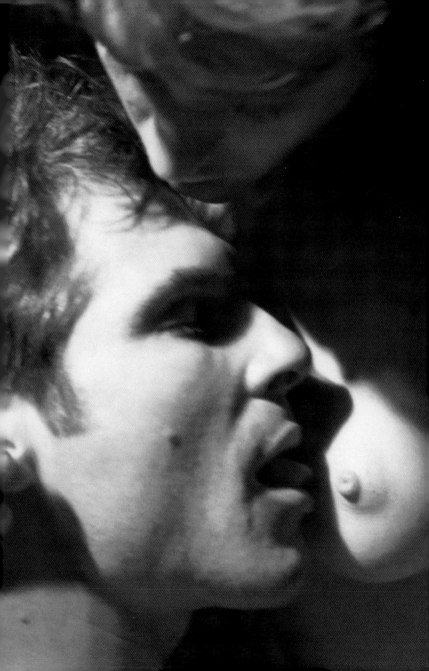

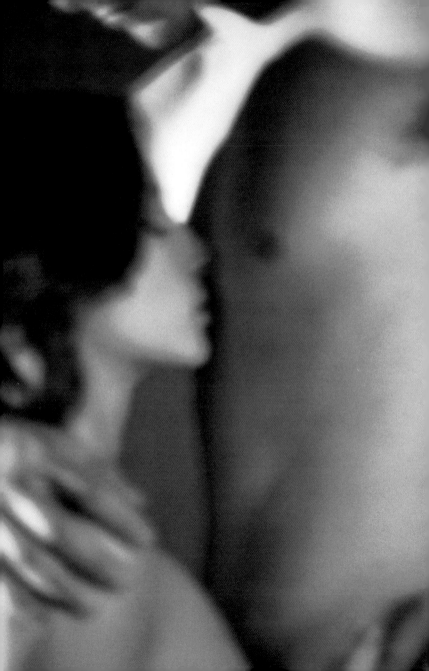

finish the fantasy...

169 As a creative writing professor, you enjoy a friend-
ly and intellectually stimulating relationship with
your students. There are two or three in your current class that are particularly bright, promising,
and attractive, and you've been working closely
with them on some special projects. One night,
you're working late in your office when your students appear at the door with what appears to be
a picnic hamper and blanket. "We wanted to show
you how much we appreciate you," the tall one
says, walking around your desk and approaching
your chair...

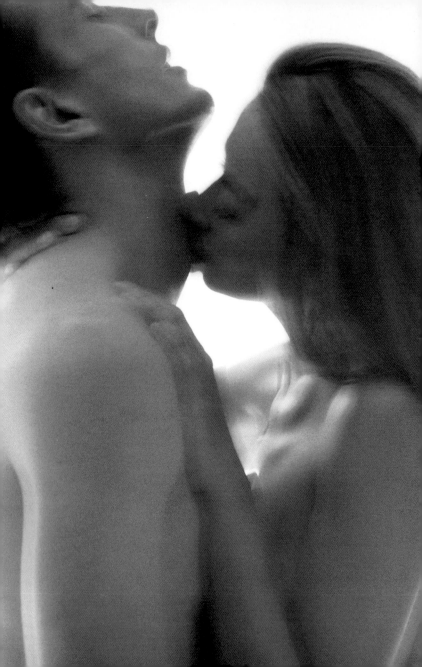

SEVEN | beyond the
bedroom

don't get caught

170 Go to your partner's workplace and find a safe place for a "quickie." If you have an office where you can lock the door, the act will still be daring but less alarming. The risk of getting caught creates an air of adventure. Use your imagination. If you like, roll a die and use the following list:

1: Boardroom
2: Boiler room
3: Deserted corridor
4: The boss's office
5: Staff room
6: Janitor's room or broom closet

171 Stimulate each other sexually while sitting in the back seat of a taxi.

172 Go to your local drive-in. Sit in the back seat and kiss and hug throughout the first movie. Make love during the second movie.

173 Go to a rock concert or crowded club wearing loose clothing and no underwear. Make love discreetly standing up in the midst of the crowd.

174 Go to your local library and find some erotic books. After a little reading gets you both hot, quietly have sex among the stacks.

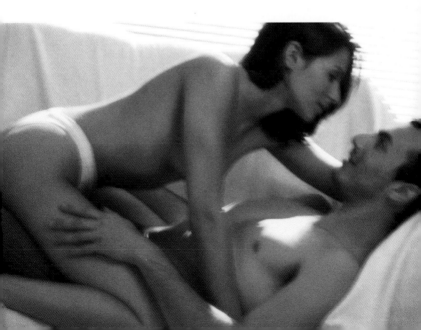

that's a new one

175   Make three lists: lovemaking techniques, unusual places to make love, and different times of day; select one from each list and carry out the instructions.

176   Try sex in a two-person tent.

177   Have sex in a swivel chair, on top of the washing machine, or on the cold kitchen floor in the morning.

178   Clear off the kitchen table and explore the fridge and cupboards for spreads, jams, butter, fruit...

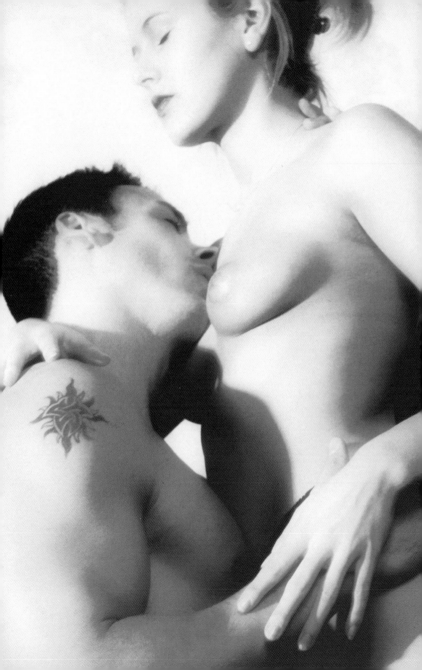

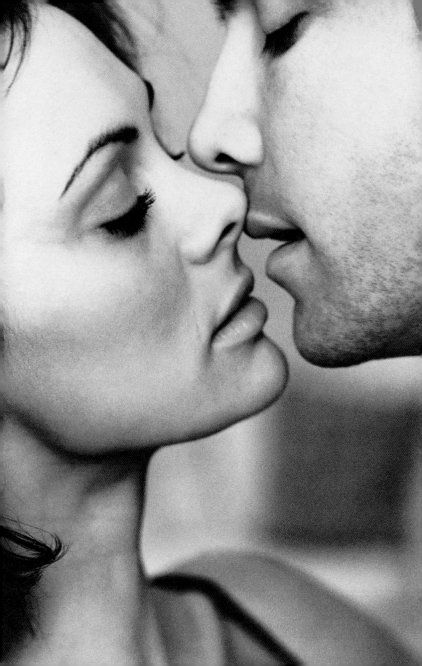

outdoor adventures

179 Learn to have sex while floating in a pool. The concentration needed to achieve this can bring you closer.

180 Have sex on a set of swings in a children's playground. (Best at night when there is no one around.)

181 Bring your lover to orgasm while on a roller coaster ride.

182 Go to your local beach or park and look for places to have sex in the fresh air.

steamy-clean fun

183 Watch your lover take a slow, pampering shower. Pretend to be a movie director and coach your lover to pay more attention to any particular area you feel they neglected.

184 Run a deep, hot bath for your lover to soak in. Become your lover's slave and cater to their every whim.

185 Pretend your partner has had a bath. Slowly dry them from the face down to the toes with a soft towel. Kiss your partner's body as you go.

186 Tie your lover's hands to the showerhead with silk scarves or hand towels. They're not allowed to say anything (gag is optional). Soap them up, massaging the creamy suds into every crevice, then rinse (preferably with a detachable, massaging showerhead). Rub them down with oil or moisturizer.

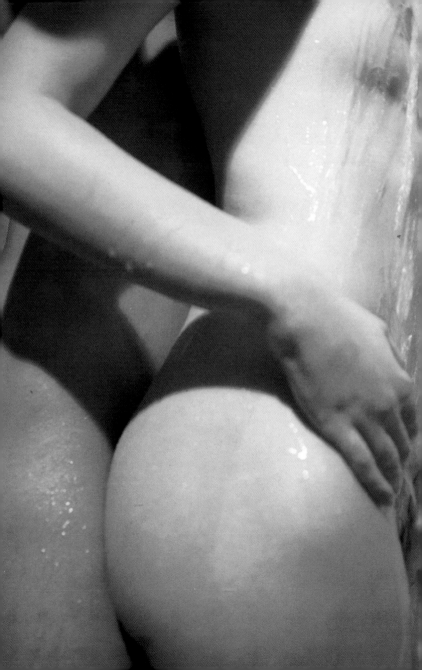

finish the fantasy...

187 You are staying in a world-class hotel. It's been a long, hard long day so you run yourself a bath, putting in luxurious bath salts. You have also arranged for the hotel to send up a masseuse. You turn off the taps and are beginning to undress when there is a knock on the door...

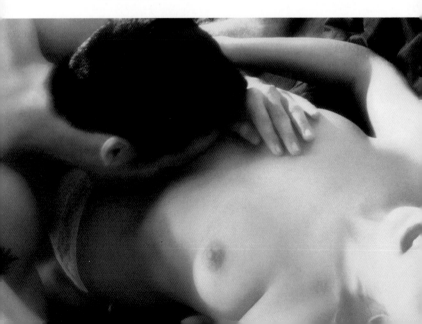

EIGHT | quiet time

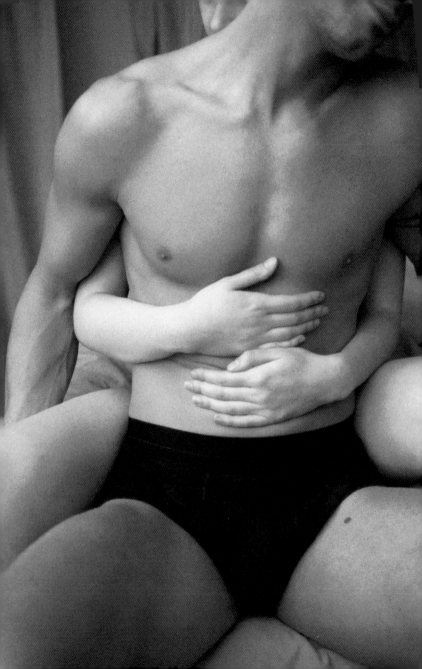

quietly intimate

188 Sit in a comfortable position facing your partner. Hold hands. Pick an intimate topic and start a conversation. One partner says the first word and then the other partner the next, taking turns until you have exhausted the topic. This becomes an exercise in mind reading and communication.

189 Sit behind your partner, one leg on either side, and gently embrace them while they lean back against you. Relax quietly in this position for several minutes. Slowly press your thumbs from the nape of your partner's neck to the base of their spine.

190 Sit cross-legged on the floor facing your partner. Rest your hands in your partner's hands, close your eyes, and breathe slowly and deeply together. Try to match each other's rhythm and mood. Do not caress or feel the need to do anything more. See how long you can stay in that position until you *have* to caress your partner.

| 9 | With your tongue, spell out action words on your lover's back for them to interpret. If they guess correctly, you must perform that action.

| 9 2 | Tap out the rhythm of a song on your lover's naked body and see if they can guess what it is. Take turns—the first to guess ten tunes has the choice of what sexual delights unfold.

| 9 3 | Use fragrant oil to write love messages on your lover's back with your finger. See if they can get the message. Try these three little symbols: I♥U

| 9 4 | Collect a variety of different objects; you can keep them in a nice cloth bag or basket. Blindfold your lover and have them guess what you are touching their naked body with. Change the pressure and speed of your stroking. Work around all parts of the body, not just the erogenous zones. Try:

- Silk scarves
- Feathers
- Straw
- Fur
- Brushes
- Gold chains

blow jobs

Blowing softly and gently on certain parts of the body can be very erotic. Find out which parts of your lover's body respond to this gentle seduction.

195 Try some of the following, then seek out your own special, sensitive areas.
- Earlobes
- Back of the neck
- Palm of the hand
- Nipples
- Inside of elbows
- Back of knees
- Inside of thighs
- Belly button

196 Moisten any erogenous area of your lover's body and blow on it with cool air from a hair dryer.

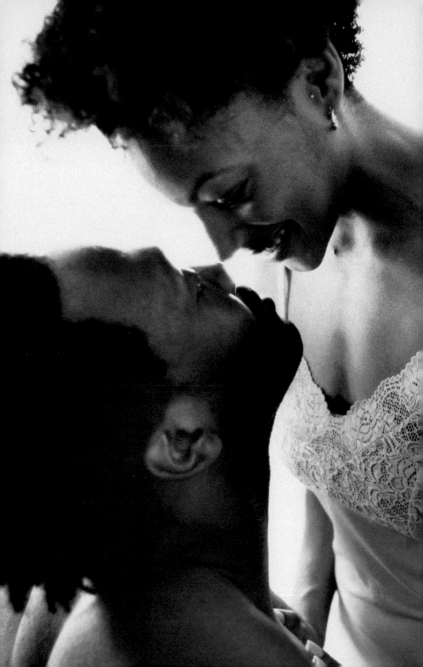

ask/tell/discuss

Read the following and ASK your partner for their view. If your partner doesn't want to talk about a particular topic, they may pass and then you can TELL them what you think. There are no right or wrong answers; the point is to DISCUSS your sexual views.

197 Seeing a naked body doesn't do anything for me.

198 Having sex without love doesn't give me pleasure.

199 It takes a lot to excite me sexually.

200 I think about sex several times a day.

201 The idea of an orgy turns me on.

202 I sometimes have a guilty conscience after sex.

203 I like to take my pleasures where I find them.

204 I've had some bad sexual experiences.

205 Watching sexy films turns me on.

rate your lover

Select the answers you identify with the most, then discuss the results with your lover.

206 How do others rate you as a lover?
a) I have to beat them away with a stick.
b) Rather well, I hope.
c) No one has complained yet.
d) Who cares?

207 Is it important to give your lover an orgasm?
a) My partner always reaches orgasm.
b) Very.
c) Not the most important thing.
d) Why? Doesn't everyone have orgasms?

208 What surfaces do you like to make love on?
a) My partner's body.
b) A mattress.
c) Soft green grass.
d) Anywhere, as long as we have fun.

209 What's the most important thing for perfect love?
a) Physical stamina
b) Imagination
c) The perfect body
d) An intelligent mind

210 Would you stop taking this quiz and make love now?
a) Yes.
b) Is this a trick question?
c) Not until I see my score.
d) Only if you promise it'll be worth it.

Scoring
(206) a=2, b=4, c=3, d=1
(207) a=3, b=4, c=2, d=1
(208) a=3, b=4, c=2, d=1
(209) a=2, b=4, c=1, d=3
(210) a=4, b=3, c=2, d=1

15–20. If you're at this end of the scale, you're a wild sex machine. You spend a lot of time thinking of and having sex. You relate well to the needs of all your different partners.

10–15. You're not up there with the great ones, but at least you try. Work on the idea that you have to give as good as you get.

5–10. Do yourself and your lover a favor and work through this book several times until you get it right.

0–5. Celibacy: Look it up in the dictionary and practice it for the rest of your life.

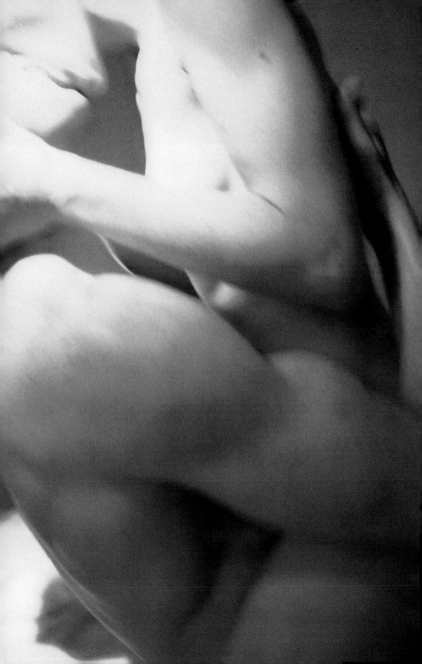

rate your lover

This quiz can be a real eye-opener. You may see yourself as the perfect lover, so compare notes and see how you rate.

211 Will your lover still be exciting at sixty-four?
a) I hope to find out.
b) I can't imagine sleeping with a wrinkly.
c) Couples don't have sex then, do they?
d) We'll keep the fire burning.

212 Can you talk to your lover about anything?
a) Yes—and it doesn't always have to make sense.
b) No—some subjects are taboo.
c) At the right time.
d) Always.

213 Does your lover lick you in all the right places?
a) I am lucky to get kisses.
b) People would pay big money for my lover's tongue.
c) When I ask.
d) It's usually, "I'll lick yours, if you lick mine."

214 Does your lover ever try new sexual things?
a) Yes—it helps keep the spice in our sex.
b) Yes—I wonder where the ideas come from.
c) We both introduce new things.
d) It's always the same.

215 Does your lover still turn your on, after all this time?
a) The flame is starting to flicker.
b) In a stronger, more mature way.
c) The physical attraction has become mental.
d) Not in the mornings.

216 Does your lover show you affection in public?
a) It comes naturally.
b) We only hold hands.
c) Our relationship doesn't work like that.
d) At the start of our relationship, but not now.

Scoring
(211) a=3, b=2, c=1, d=4
(212) a=4, b=1, c=2, d=3
(213) a=1, b=4, c=3, d=2
(214) a=3, b=2, c=4, d=1
(215) a=1, b=4, c=3, d=2
(216) a=4, b=3, c=2, d=1

18–24. Wow! Your lover is the type people fantasize about.

12–18. Sex and romance are working well. Don't let things slip and you'll reap the rewards forever.

6–12. Sounds like your lover is a few condoms short of a full pack. Don't give up, use more positive, lusty suggestions and you never know what might come.

0–6. Pack and leave now. With all the people in the world, you both deserve better.

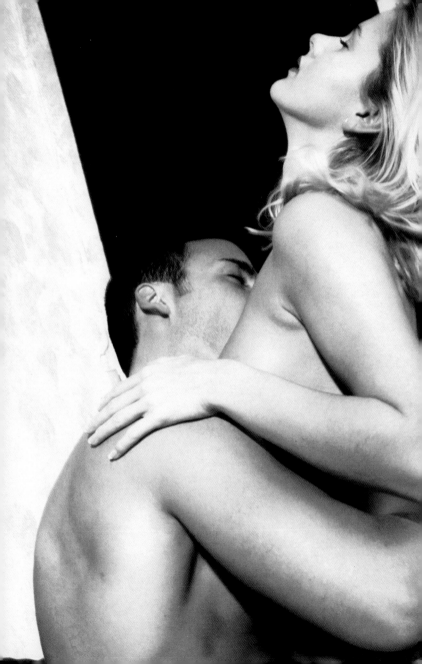

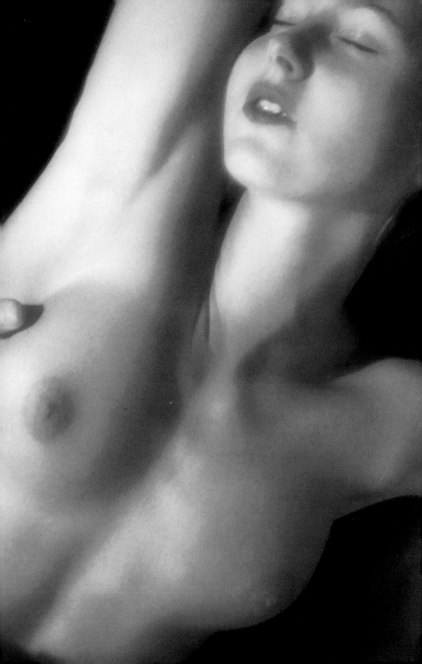

finish the fantasy...

217 It's a warm and sultry night. You are lying on the bed naked. The lights are out and the moonlight is shining through the window. You feel hot and horny; beads of sweat form on your body. The French windows are open and a gentle breeze blows the curtains aside. A figure is standing at the door...

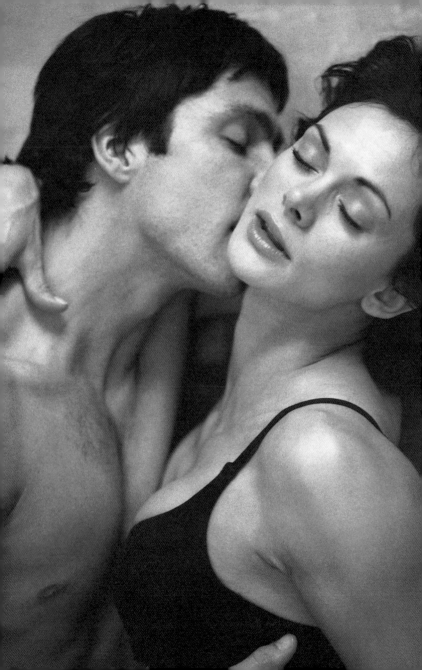

NINE | the world of imagination

designer sex

2|8 Design a sexual technique or new sexual position you have not heard of before and name it after your-selves.

2|9 Invent a technique, create a story, or organize a bawdy evening that will make your partner reach an orgasm without being touched.

220 Make a list of sexy ideas and whisper them into your lover's ear. Ask your lover to rate the ideas on a scale of one to ten.

22| Research sexual techniques from different cultures and religions.

222 Imagine any part of your lover's body as a warm, juicy peach or mango. Take your time as you devour it.

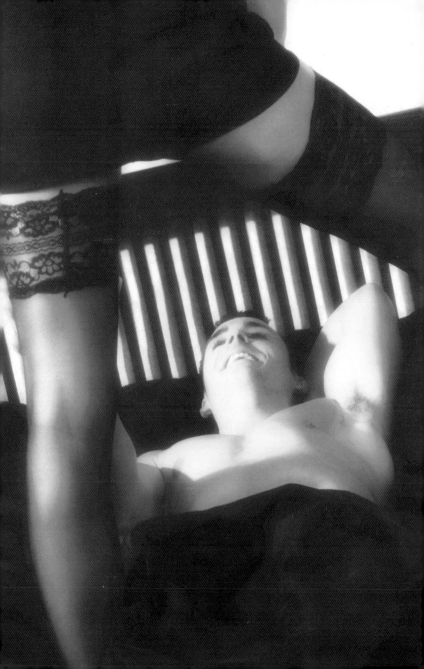

if you could...

Talk about your answers and try out (or approximate) as many as you like. Use as a basis for role-playing or dress up.

223 If you could bathe in a deep bath filled with the liquid of your choice, what would it be?

224 If you could get the perfect massage, what would it be like?

225 If you could live anywhere in the world, where would it be?

226 If you could live in any time period, when would it be? Who would you be?

227 If you could choose a lover of any race or nationality, what would they look like?

228 If you could snap your fingers and change your appearance, what would you look like?

229 If you could talk about any subject, no matter how taboo, what would it be?

230 If you could star in a porno movie, what role would you play? What's the plot?

231 If you could give your lover anything, what would it be?

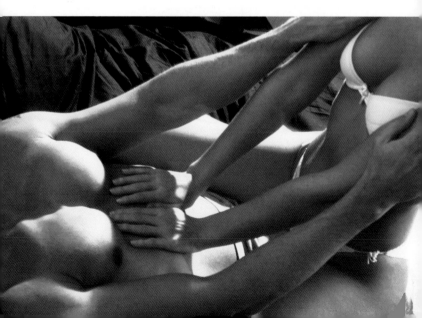

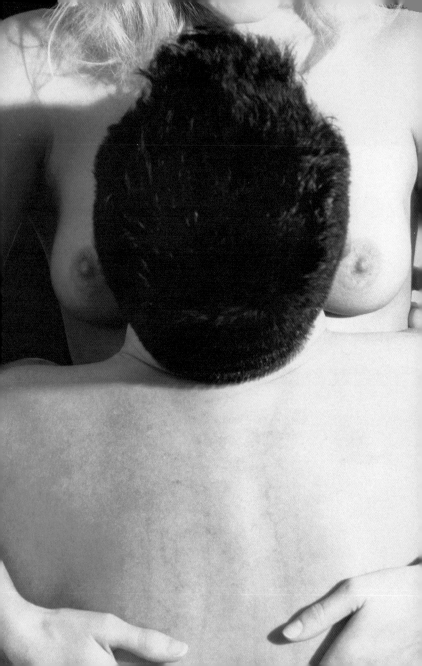

talking heads

Imagine your various body parts can talk—ask for what they want, say what mood they are in, express likes and dislikes— what would they say?

232 If your vagina could talk, how would she say she is feeling right now?

233 If your penis could talk, where would he want to be?

234 If your breasts could talk, what would they request?

235 If your hands could talk, what would they say they want to do?

236 Is there a neglected body part that would like to ask for attention?

love potion #9

The Ancient Greeks and Romans were probably the first to take love potions seriously, but it was the influence of witchcraft in the mid-sixteenth century that sparked spells of love in other parts of the world.

237 Prepare a love spell or love potion to drive your lover mad with desire. Share the contents of the spell with your lover.

238 Try this charm based on an old Austrian folk tale using an apple. Write a sexy invitation on nice paper and tear in half. Place half by your front door (or, if you're feeling extra lucky, behind your bedroom door). Place the other half in your bosom. If you think about the one you love positively, then at the stroke of midnight, your lover will be standing at your door.

239 Take hold of your lover's hand and caress it gently. Read their palm—with a positive outlook.

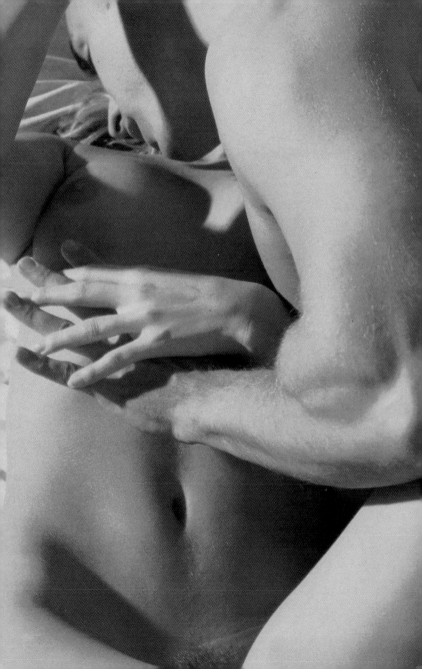

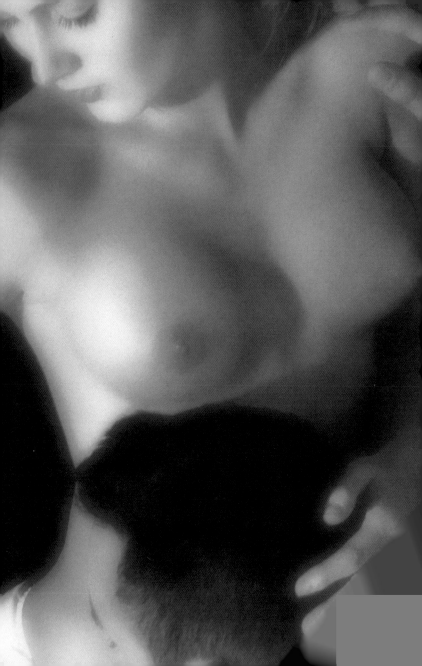

treasure hunt

240 Using a dab of honey, make an "x" somewhere on your body for your lover to find just using their tongue.

241 Using your tongue, map out the places on your lover's body that are sweet, bitter, salty, and sour.

242 Place a sweet sauce on the left nipple and a hot or sour sauce on the right nipple. Toss a coin to see which nipple your lover is to suck on first.

243 Use washable ink pens to draw treasure maps on your own or each other's bodies. Follow the map to the treasure.

you're stranded on a desert island...

244   With your partner, make up a survival kit that you'd want to have on a desert island. Spend the weekend pretending you're stranded.

Discuss the following questions with your lover. Describe in detail the sexiest fantasy you can invent.

245   In what exotic place would you like to make love?

246   If you were stranded on a desert island, who (apart from your partner) would you like to be there with you?

247   What reading material would you like to have with you?

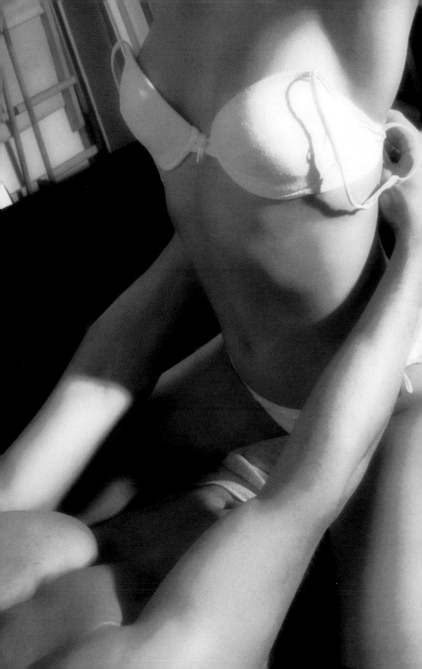

248 I awoke naked and alone on a desert island. All I could see was the ocean, masses of palm trees...and footprints in the sand. Were these the prints of an unfriendly native? Should I seek refuge among the palm trees or should I follow the footprints? I decided to follow the footprints. In a matter minutes, the prints led me to a hut with a thatch roof. Slowly, I walked toward the hut and through the door-way. In the dim light of the interior, I saw...

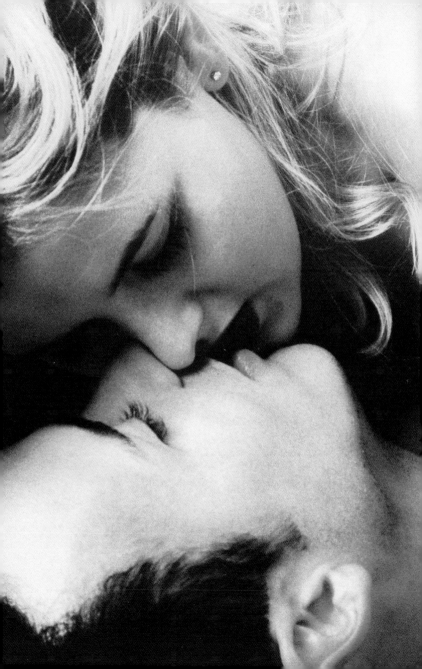

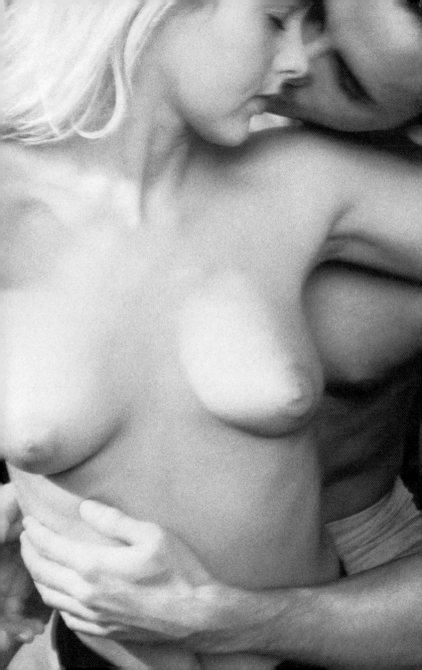

TEN | classics with a twist

2 4 9 Play Spin the Bottle and add foreplay other than kissing.

2 5 0 Play "sexual truth or dare" together.

2 5 1 Play naked Twister.

2 5 2 Play ping-pong in your sexiest underwear. A little paddling is allowed.

2 5 3 Play strip-dice. Take turns rolling the dice and the one with the lowest number has to seductively remove a piece of clothing.

2 5 4 Have a two-legged race. Tape or tie each other's legs together and try having sex.

2 5 5 Play strip poker, but start by taking underwear off first.

2 5 6 Play naked statues and see who can hold still longer.

257 Stand naked in front of each other. Become mirror images and mime each other's movements.

258 Play zoo and pretend you're the animal of your choice. Make love as that animal. Be as wild, or sleek, or slippery as you like.

259 Play submarine by performing oral sex in a full bathtub.

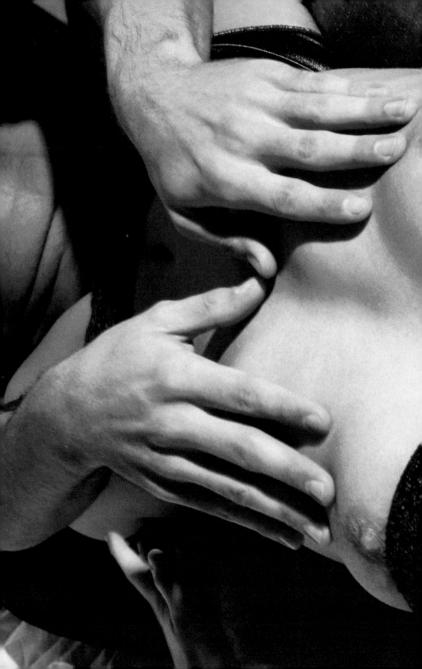

getting naked

260 Try ripping each other's clothes off before sex. Wear old clothes especially for the occasion.

261 Undress each other using just your feet and toes.

262 Blindfold each other, then undress each other slowly and sensuously, touching and caressing each part of the body as it is revealed to your hands.

263 Put on some raunchy stripper music and gyrate your body to the beat. As you shed each garment, throw the clothes toward your lover. You might want to start off wearing tassels or other appropriately tacky items. When you're naked, jump them unceremoniously.

264 Put on some exotic belly dancing music and do a teasing, graceful strip.

kama sutra games

The Kama Sutra provides both a way of approaching sex with attention and open-mindedness, and a catalog of sexual positions, some quite exotic. Exploring the Kama Sutra will help you find new freedom and playfulness in your lovemaking. Any number of English translations are available.

265 Play Kama Sutra bingo. The winner gets to choose the position.

266 Make up your own Kama Sutra photo album with numbered photos. Pick a number, or close your eyes and point to a page to see what position to achieve.

267 Make up a cardboard cube and stick on six photos of your favorite Kama Sutra positions. Roll the cube and spend a few minutes in the position before rolling the cube again to continue.

268 Have playing cards made up depicting the two of you in different Kama Sutra positions, with two copies of each position. Play "Go Fish." The winner earns sex in their favorite position.

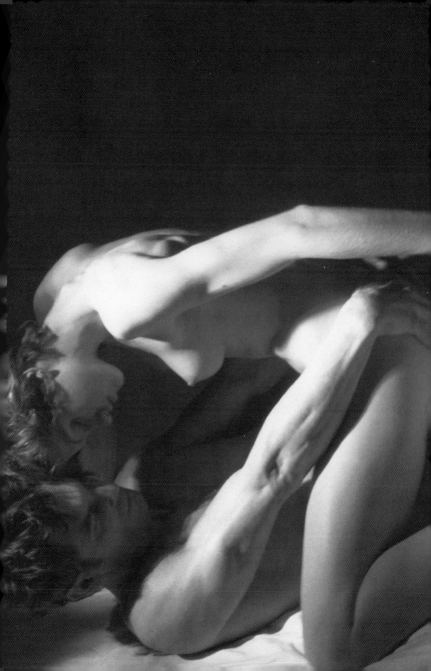

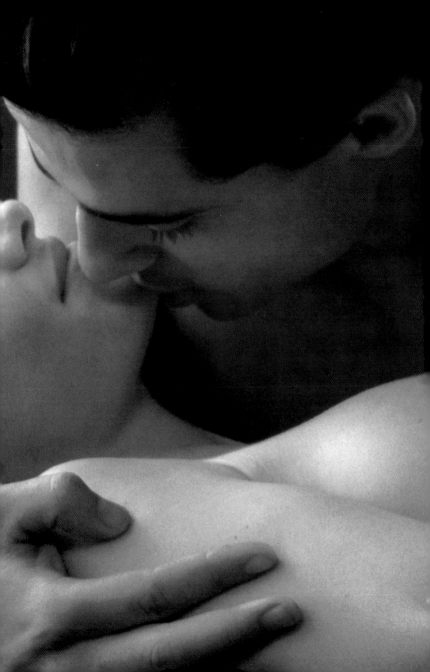

269 You are staying at a beautiful resort in the mountains for the weekend. Your companion cancelled at the last minute, so you have the canopied king-size bed and fireplace all to yourself. Swimming in the lake, you notice the lithe body and healthy tan of another guest who appears to be unaccompanied. Later, down by the stables, the same stranger catches you in a quiet corner...

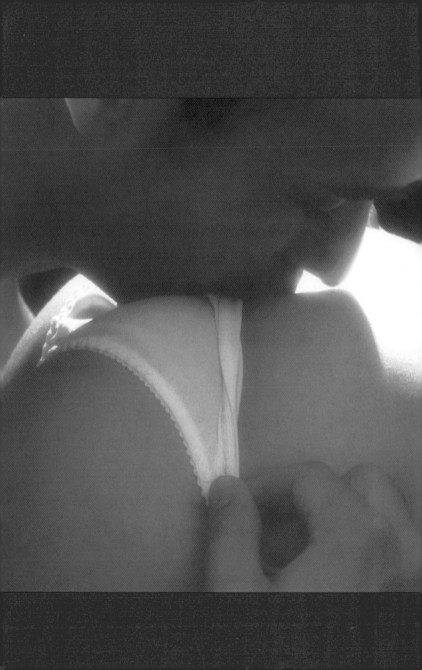

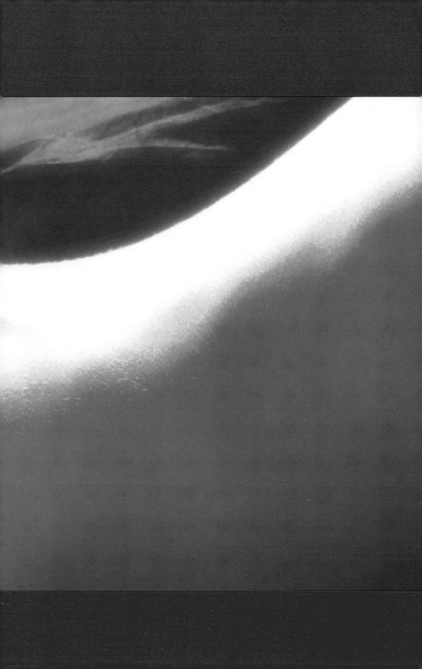

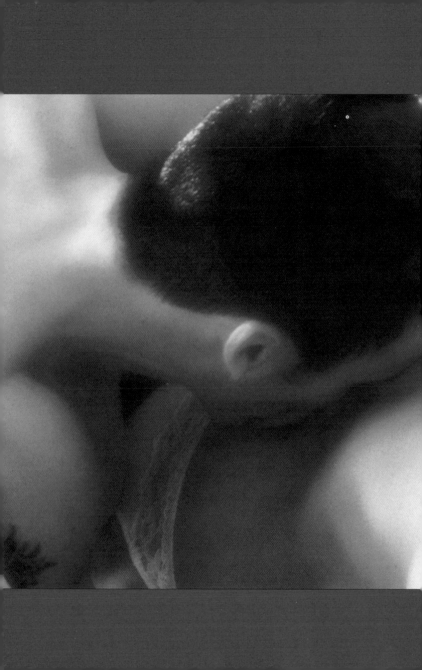

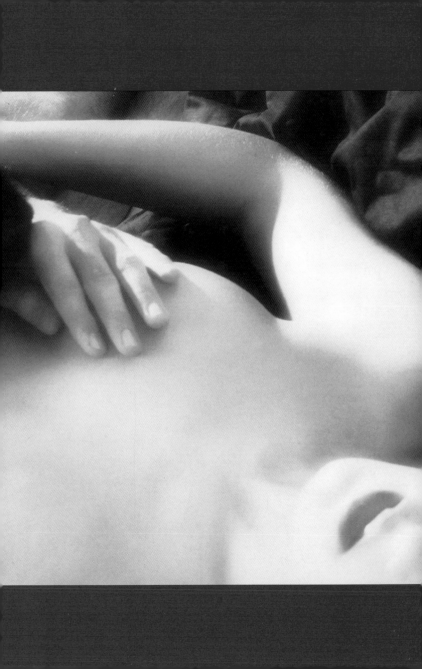

about the author

Hugh de Beer is the creator of the popular *Foreplay*® board game (over 200,000 sold). He has written five books, which are bestsellers in Australia, where he lives and works.